Diabetic Neurop .

Symptoms, Treatments, Diet, Management, Natural Remedies, Vitamins and Exercises all covered.

by

Robert Rymore

Published by IMB Publishing 2014

Table Of Contents

Table of Contents

Table of Contents

Table of Contents

Foreword

According to statistics from the World Health Organization, a staggering 370 million people worldwide have diabetes; sadly the number of patients being diagnosed with the disease looks set to continue, and some experts have described diabetes as an "epidemic".

As the cases of diabetes continue to rise, so do the chances of developing one of the many complications that are associated with it.

The most common complications of diabetes – and one of the most disabling and painful complications – is diabetic neuropathy.

As it stands now, diabetic neuropathy is not curable and treatments that will help alleviate all of the symptoms have so far proven evasive.

However, as you'll learn throughout this book, there is plenty that a patient can do to help themselves; throughout the book patients will find many methods of making their symptoms more manageable.

This book will put the power into your hands and help you to realise that despite the lack of treatments available, much can still be done to reduce pain, find support groups, and gain control of your diabetes.

Introduction

It is estimated that up to 40% of diabetics have one of the most common complications of diabetes: diabetic neuropathy. Patients can be affected by diabetic neuropathy to a greater or a lesser degree and the symptoms of neuropathy can become severe in some patients, causing pain and disability.

Diabetic neuropathy affects patients with both type one and type two diabetes; the longer a person has had diabetes, the more likely they are to develop neuropathy. The pain and disability that can come with neuropathy can be hard to cope with at times, however, there are ways of managing this painful nerve condition and there are ways of helping to prevent it, all of which will be discussed later on in the book.

This book aims to provide a management guide to help anyone who is living with this condition. It will outline treatments, both medical and natural, give practical advice to help alleviate some of the most distressing symptoms of neuropathy, such as pain and the burning and tingling sensations that are common to nerve damage, and will highlight the symptoms so that you know what to look out for and what to do if you notice any of the warning signs of neuropathy.

While neuropathy is a common complication of diabetes, it is also preventable in many cases. So this book will explore how patients can help themselves to avoid this complication of diabetes and will also examine some of the other causes of neuropathy, and detail the treatments available.

Chapter 1) Diabetic Neuropathy

1) What is Diabetic Neuropathy?

Neuropathy is a disease or disorder of the nerves. "Neuro" refers to the nerves or nervous system, while "pathy" is Greek in origin and means suffering or disease.

While there are many different causes of neuropathy, diabetes is a major contributor, due to the high concentrations of glucose that can cause damage to the nerves.

The damage is most often caused to the peripheral nerves and primarily affects the hands and feet. However, some diabetics can also go on to develop autonomic neuropathy – a form of neuropathy that affects the autonomic nervous system, as well as other forms of the nerve disease. This is a subject that will be explored later on in the book.

What is Motor Neuropathy?

Motor Neuropathy- definition

Motor neuropathy refers to the damage done to the motor nerves; the motor nerves are responsible for controlling movement. These nerves can be damaged through diabetes due to high blood glucose levels.

Once the motor nerves become damaged, walking can become difficult. Patients might also begin to experience muscle wasting in their arms or legs, or both. Motor nerve neuropathy can also cause other symptoms, such as muscle spasms, restless legs, and cramps, which can cause painful contractions in the lower leg muscles.

Motor neuropathies can also have many other causes, some of which will be discussed later.

Motor Neuropathy -Treatment

The treatment of motor neuropathy in diabetics involves controlling pain, maintaining mobility and addressing any problems a patient might have with their blood glucose control.

Once a patient has got their glucose levels under control, they are likely to see a reduction in their symptoms; further damage to the nerves is also preventable by keeping the blood sugars well balanced.

Is There a Cure for Neuropathy?

Unfortunately, there is no cure for diabetic peripheral neuropathy; it is more a matter of managing the symptoms.. However, controlling your glucose levels will go a long way to reducing the symptoms of neuropathy, such as tingling and pain. Surgery can help some patients but a lot of research needs to be done on this

Some of the symptoms can also be successfully managed by discussing with your doctor the best kind of pain medication for your condition. Medications such as paracetamol and ibuprofen aren't usually effective for coping with the nerve pain that comes with neuropathy, so your doctor might discuss trying you out on an anti-depressant medication called amitriptyline, or something similar, as these kinds of anti-depressants can also be effective at helping reduce nerve pain.

If your pain is severe, then you might be referred to a pain clinic to help you find ways of managing your neuropathy more effectively.

2) Diabetic Neuropathy - Symptoms

The first sign that something is wrong is often a tingling in the hands or feet. This may be a minor irritation at first, and may only occur occasionally; however, if the problem is allowed to continue, then it could worsen. Diabetic neuropathy is a condition worth addressing as soon as possible before the symptoms have a chance to progress.

Pain might also feel like electrical shocks running along your feet, or your feet might just feel uncomfortable to touch. Some people become so sensitive that they can't even tolerate a blanket near their legs and feet, but this is only in severe cases.

Patients with the early stages of neuropathy might also notice numbness in their hands or feet. This might only be minor to begin with, but it can worsen as time goes on.

People with diabetic neuropathy might also develop problems with walking, and in advanced cases might go on to develop foot problems such as ulcers or deformities of their feet. If this is the case, you should be referred to an Orthotist who will help fit some orthotics to make walking more comfortable, and to give some protection to your feet when you walk.

If the muscles become very tight, then it might also be recommended that you wear night splints. If these are suggested then they will usually be provided by the hospital, but patients should make sure that splints do not rub against their skin. If they do, then ask your specialist if they can do anything to address these issues.

While this book mainly concentrates on the subject of diabetic peripheral neuropathy and its symptoms, there are several diabetic neuropathies; you'll find details of these on the following pages.

Diagnosis

If you have very obvious signs of diabetic neuropathy, then your doctor is likely to be able to diagnose your condition by looking over your medical history and assessing your symptoms.

In some cases, they might carry out some tests, such as the filament test. You might also be referred to see a neurologist at your local hospital where they would carry out nerve conduction tests and electromyography tests to monitor how well your nerves are working.

These tests involve having a sensor attached to your arm. Although these tests are not painful, you are likely to feel some mild discomfort while the tests are being carried out. The assessments only take a few moments, and your consultant will then be able to give you the results and explain more to you about how well your nerves are working.

You could also be asked if you have experienced any signs of muscle weakness and the consultant might test your reflexes. The consultant might also discuss motor and sensory function with you as this can sometimes be affected by diabetic neuropathy. In case you are unclear what this means, motor function refers to how our muscles move while sensory refers to our ability to feel cold, heat, pain etc.

You might also be asked to undergo further tests that will involve touching your feet with a pin or you might be asked to close your eyes and your doctor will use something light like a feather and ask you to tell him when you feel it touch against your skin. This is a way of testing the sensory function and how well you are able to feel your feet.

Dr Bonnie Gerecke is board certified in Neurology and Neurological Medicine and is Chief of the Division of Neurology and Medical Director of Rehabilitation at the Mercy Medical Center in Baltimore. In the following pages, Dr Gerecke explains some of the other types of neuropathy that can affect diabetics.

Peripheral neuropathy is damage or disease affecting the nerves. About 30-50 percent of patients with diabetes mellitus develop peripheral neuropathy. Symptoms of diabetic neuropathy are diverse and include numbness and tingling in the hands and feet, burning pain, and weakness. There are several different types of diabetic neuropathy including the following: diabetic sensorimotor polyneuropathy (DSP), painful small fiber neuropathy (SFN), diabetic lumbosacral polyradiculoneuropathy (DLSPRN), thoracic radiculopathy, focal mononeuropathies, and autonomic neuropathy. A patient can have one or more of these conditions at any time. Diabetic neuropathy can be mild and asymptomatic (only discovered on examination by a physician, for example) or can be severe and debilitating. The duration of time that the patient has diabetes and the level of hyperglycemia are, for the most part, directly correlated with an increased risk of developing diabetic neuropathy, with few exceptions. The pathogenesis of diabetic neuropathy is likely to be multifactorial. It could be due to a combination of genetic factors predisposing a person to develop this condition as well as environmental ones, such as total hyperglycemic exposure, smoking, and ethanol ingestion, among others.

3) Diabetic sensorimotor polyneuropathy

Diabetic sensorimotor polyneuropathy (DSP) is the most common form of diabetic neuropathy. Patients with this condition most commonly experience numbness and tingling- starting in the toes and then spreading to involve the feet. It can gradually ascend the legs and then can involve the hands. Patients with this condition often complain that they feel like their legs are "wrapped in tight bandages" or that it feels like there is "water running down the legs." In more severe cases of this form of neuropathy, patients can develop weakness, predominantly in the feet. They may develop foot drops, which occur when there is weakness in the distal muscles of the legs and the foot slaps on the ground due to weakness.

4) Small-Fiber neuropathy

Another form of diabetic neuropathy is small-fiber neuropathy (SFN). This condition is due to nerve damage to the very small nerve fibers, particularly in the feet. Patients describe severe burning pain in their feet. They experience allodynia, which is the sensation that a non-noxious stimulus is painful. For example, they cannot tolerate having bed sheets cover their feet at night and cannot walk barefoot on a cold floor because this is too painful. There is no weakness associated with this condition. However, it is very painful and can be extremely disabling.

5) Focal mononeuropathies

Patients with diabetic neuropathy are also predisposed to develop what are called focal mononeuropathies. These neuropathies include median neuropathies (carpal tunnel syndrome), ulnar neuropathies (nerve damage at the elbow), and peroneal neuropathies (damage to the nerve just below the knee). These conditions can also occur in non-diabetics but patients with diabetes have an increased risk of developing them. The exact reason for this predilection is uncertain, but it may be that they are more susceptible to compressive injuries. Diabetic patients also have an increased risk of developing cranial mononeuropathies. The cranial nerves are the nerves that emerge directly from the brain and innervate muscles of the face and internal organs. There are 12 cranial nerves. Patients with diabetes have an increased risk of developing damage to the 6th and 3rd cranial nerves, causing eye movement abnormalities. This may be due to ischemia to the nerves, although this is not certain.

6) Diabetic lumbosacral polyradiculoneuropathy

Diabetic lumbosacral polyradiculoneuropathy (DLSPRN) is a less common form of neuropathy than DSP but is more fulminant in its onset and the degree with which it affects patients. It is also unique in that this condition tends to affect diabetic patients who have good control of their blood sugar levels compared to the other forms of neuropathy, which are usually more prevalent in those who have poorly controlled diabetes. The classic presentation of DLSPRN is one in which the patient develops an abrupt onset of severe pain, often in the thigh and upper leg, followed by severe muscle atrophy, weakness, and often tingling in the leg. It is usually unilateral but can also be bilateral. There is often weight-loss and overall malaise associated with this condition. Patients are often misdiagnosed with a disc herniation in the lower back and some even undergo unnecessary spine surgery because of this misdiagnosis. DLSPRN is a self-remitting condition and patients often hit a nadir in terms of weakness before they start to experience an improvement in strength. Some patients make a full recovery but many patients have chronic irreversible nerve damage and weakness.

7) Diabetic thoracic radiculopathy

Diabetic thoracic radiculopathy is a condition that typically occurs in middle aged individuals with diabetes. It is heralded by an abrupt onset of severe neuropathic burning pain radiating around the chest from the back, often unilaterally. There is hypersensitivity to touch on the skin of the area involved, and sometimes there may be out pouching of the abdominal wall at the level of pain due to muscle weakness. There is often associated weight loss. Diabetic thoracic radiculopathy can be confused for an intra-abdominal process and like patients with DLSPRN; patients with this condition often undergo unnecessary testing and even surgery for a possible intra-abdominal lesion. Diabetic thoracic radiculopathy is self-remitting, although it can be very painful during the throes of the illness.

Diabetic autonomic neuropathy is another form of neuropathy that occurs most commonly in patients with poorly controlled diabetes. Patients with autonomic neuropathy due to diabetes often also have DSP, although it can also be present as an isolated phenomenon. The autonomic nervous system regulates the internal organs of the body. Autonomic nervous system dysfunction can cause unexplained tachycardia, orthostatic hypotension, poor exercise tolerance, gastroparesis, erectile dysfunction, bladder dysfunction, hyperhydrosis (excessive sweating), and many other symptoms. It can be debilitating and at its worst, life threatening, when patients develop cardiac arrthymias or inability to perceive pain from cardiac ischemia due to nerve damage.

8) Definition - Neuropathic Pain

Neuropathic pain refers to nerve pain. This kind of pain often arises when the nerve signals aren't functioning properly. If you feel burning, shooting or stabbing pains or tingling then this would be described as neuropathic pain.

Neuropathic pain can also refer to the type of pain that people feel when they suffer from a painful condition such as neuralgia, or nerve pain that is felt in the face.

9) What is peripheral neuropathic pain?

The term peripheral neuropathic pain simply refers to the pain and strange sensations such as stabbing and tingling pain that are felt in the hands and feet in patients with diabetic neuropathy.

This type of pain is often a sure sign that there is something wrong with the way the nerves are functioning, so as soon as you start to experience symptoms like this, then you need to seek medical attention.

For information on the various treatments for neuropathic pain, please read on to the next section.

10) Diabetic Neuropathy - Treatment

Unfortunately, there are no conventional diabetic neuropathy treatments as such. When it comes to the treatment of diabetic neuropathy, the emphasis tends to be on controlling pain and discomfort, using orthotics to make walking more comfortable, and in advanced stages, if you have damage caused to your joints because of the neuropathy, then surgery may be discussed to help fix this. Although the treatment of diabetic peripheral neuropathy isn't easy, there are many options available, as you'll discover as you read the book.

People often react differently to painkillers, so finding a medication that is effective for you will be a matter of trial and error. You'll need to discuss with your doctor which method of pain control he feels is best for you. However, the following pages will outline some of the most commonly prescribed painkillers used as treatment for diabetic peripheral neuropathy.

If you are prescribed a medication to be taken just once a day, then it is often advised that it is taken at night time. This is because pain is often worse at night. However, if you experience a lot of pain during the day time hours as well, talk to your doctor about taking a medication that can be used twice a day so you can control pain during both the day time and the night time.

11) Anti-depressants

When it comes to controlling pain, anti-depressants are often prescribed, as these have been found to be effective at controlling nerve pain. Anti-depressants also make a suitable treatment for diabetic neuropathy.

Medications that you might be prescribed include Amitriptyline or Nortriptiline. It should be noted that as with all medications, anti-depressants are not without their side effects, however, most people will find these side effects pretty minor and if they don't affect your everyday life and help you to manage your symptoms, then this may well be the best course of treatment for you.

12) Anti- Epilepsy Medication

Another form of treatment for managing neuropathy pain is drugs that are used to control seizures; Neurontin and Lyrica are two of the drugs commonly prescribed for nerve pain. Lyrica is a drug that is often prescribed to help control anxiety disorders and OCD, but it can also be an effective means of pain management for some people.

Although it is an effective pain reliever, Neurontin can cause some undesirable side effects such as dizziness and tiredness. There can also be some other side effects with this type of medication. Although the worst of the side effects are often rare, it is best to discuss this with your doctor if you are concerned.

Lyrica, which is also known as Pregbalin, can also have some unwanted side effects. It can cause drowsiness and dizziness, as well as a dry mouth and problems concentrating. Pregbalin is often prescribed to help counter neuropathic pain so it is often suggested to help patients with discomfort caused by their diabetic neuropathy pain.

Pregbalin can also have some more serious side effects in some patients and if you are already prone to depressive thoughts, then taking this type of medication is something that you'll need to discuss carefully with the person in charge of your medical care.

If you are prescribed this type of medication, it is likely that you will be told to take it up to three times a day. Some doctors suggest taking the medication last thing at night to help relieve any night time discomfort caused by your diabetic neuropathy.

13) Lidocaine

Lidocaine is a local anaesthetic and helps alleviate pain by numbing the affected area. Lidocaine is often applied in the form of patches, but it can also be bought as a cream. If your doctor doesn't prescribe it, Lidocaine creams can be bought online and it is available over the counter as well, however, it is a good idea to speak to your consultant before trying this type of treatment.

Lidocaine does have some side effects, as do most other medications, but Lidocaine can be extremely effective for nerve pain when taken correctly.

As always, you should discuss any concerns you have over medications you have been prescribed with your doctor. They are the person best placed to know how to help you, and whether they think that this type of medication will be effective for your neuropathy pain.

Some people find that they get a burning pain when they apply the cream, while others find that the patches can cause some skin irritation, if this is a problem for you, then speak to your doctor about alternative means of pain control.

14) Tramadol

Tramadol is usually prescribed for pain that is considered moderately severe or severe. Tramadol is from the opioid group of medications and is available in pill, injection form, as a liquid solution, a soluble solution, and in many other forms. It is commonly prescribed for the control of nerve pain and it also has anti-depressant properties.

Possible side effects include headaches, constipation, nausea, dry mouth, drowsiness and fatigue. There can also be some more severe side effects, but these are rare. If any of the side effects of any of your prescribed medications concern you – and if you feel the side effects are more severe than the symptoms they are meant to control – then speak to your doctor/physician for advice.

Tramadol is sold as Dramadol in the UK.

15) Is peripheral neuropathy reversible?

There is a bit of a question mark over whether or not neuropathy can be reversed. Some experts argue that neuropathy can't be reversed, while others state reversing peripheral neuropathy is possible. As stated earlier on in the book, there certainly is no cure for neuropathy, but you might be able to address some of the issues that contribute to it.

If your neuropathy was caused by a vitamin deficiency such as vitamin B12, then once that has been corrected, you are likely to see a reduction in the symptoms. However, once nerves are damaged, it is hard to repair them, and if your nerve damage has occurred over a long period of time then it will be even more difficult to reverse neuropathy or to reduce the symptoms.

Diabetic neuropathy and hereditary neuropathies cannot be reversed according to some experts, but if you look around on forums you will see many diabetics stating that their neuropathy has been reversed due to better glucose control.

However, it is more likely that the symptoms have just been reduced, and if symptoms can be reduced to such an extent that some people feel their neuropathy has vanished, then it shows that there is plenty that can be done by patients to help themselves.

Another factor to take into consideration is the length of time you have had the symptoms. The longer you have had neuropathy, the less chance there is of being able to reverse it.

If you are a type two diabetic, then the damage to your nerves could have occurred over a long period of time and you might not have realised that some of the symptoms you were experiencing were down to nerve damage. If this is the case, your best approach is to get your glucose levels under control and see if you can reduce the symptoms that way.

When it comes to coping with neuropathy, your best hope is to take action to address the symptoms and deal with any underlying issues that could be making your symptoms worse.

Many patients with diabetic neuropathy can also get some reduction in their symptoms by taking various vitamin supplements and trying complimentary therapies.

While different people will see different results, it is worth trying some of these therapies to see if they can make your symptoms more manageable.

So, while it is not likely that you can see a complete reversal of your symptoms, it is likely that by following the practical advice laid out in the chapters ahead you can at least begin to find some effective ways of managing your painful neuropathy symptoms.

There are plenty of suggestions detailed throughout the book, and while none of them promise a reversal of your neuropathy, they do offer at least some relief from some of the more uncomfortable symptoms. You'll find a chapter on vitamin therapy and supplements that might be useful to you in the next chapter. If pain isn't your main issue, but you've found yourself struggling to maintain dexterity, then you'll find a chapter filled with practical advice later on in the book.

If you read on, you'll also discover advice on natural pain relievers, managing night time pain and lowering your blood glucose levels, and all of these things will make living with neuropathy much easier.

Chapter 2) Vitamins for Neuropathy

When it comes to neuropathy treatment, many people feel that vitamins can be effective at helping to combat at least some of the discomfort.

While many patients feel that they have benefits from taking supplements for their neuropathy, there isn't an awful lot of data available that supports just how effective they are as forms of treatment. Studies into the many alternative treatments are often small, so they don't always give a clear idea of how well they could work.

That being said, vitamins and minerals are usually affordable to buy, and if there are few other options available then they are worth a try; some people claim that they have seen a reversal of their neuropathy through taking various supplements.

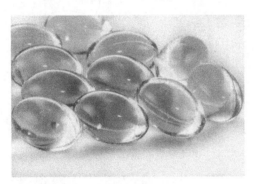

1) Benfotiamine

Benfotiamine is a fat soluble form of vitamin B1. This supplement is believed to be one of the most beneficial to diabetics, as it is thought that taking it in capsule form can help to prevent some of the complications of diabetes. It is also thought to help lower the requirements for insulin and to better help control blood glucose levels.

In recent years, there have been many encouraging studies surrounding this supplement and there are many testimonies available from people with diabetes and diabetic neuropathy who will attest to effectiveness of taking benfotiamine. It is believed that this form of Vitamin B1 protects the body from glycation, thus protecting diabetics from the more serious types of complications.

The supplement is readily available and is extremely cost effective so this might be the supplement of choice for many diabetics. A study by the 2nd Department of Internal Medicine, Municipal St. John's Hospital, Budapest, found that benfotiamine was most effective when taken in higher doses. Participants in the study were given 320mg a day, and were given the capsules in four separate doses throughout the day.

The study detailed above is just one of many detailing the benefits of benfotiamine supplementation.

2) Methylcobalamin

Some studies into the use of methylcobalamin for the treatment of diabetic neuropathy have been inconclusive. However, many diabetics do feel that they get some relief through taking this supplement.

The same studies have also shown that while patients might not have reported an improvement in their symptoms, there were no noticeable side effects.

Methylcobalamin is a form of vitamin B12 and is believed to be better absorbed and better tolerated when taken this way. It is available in tablet form, and depending on the brand, it is suggested that it be taken every two – four days.

In a recent study carried out by Jacqueline C. Dominguez, Arlene R. Ng, Ludwig F. Damian, and published in the JDM journal, it was shown that patients had an improvement in symptoms, such as ataxia and tingling; pinprick sensation and vibration sensation were also improved. However, the participants in the study were given large doses of methylcobalamin; doses of 1500 μgm were given daily over a six week period and the study was carried out with patients suffering from polyneuropathy.

3) B Vitamins

B Vitamins in general are thought to be good for neuropathy; however, some of the studies have proved to be inconclusive. Some studies have determined that taking high doses of B complex vitamins can help reduce the intensity of painful neuropathy, while others report a reduction in numbness.

Certainly, a lack of some B vitamins can cause some forms of neuropathy. Vegetarians can develop neuropathy due to a lack of vitamin B12 in their diet. However, what many studies don't show is whether the patients were deficient in B vitamins in the first place, if they were, it might just mean that supplementing with B complex vitamins corrected the underlying deficiency, thus easing some of the symptoms of neuropathy.

Too much of some B vitamins can also contribute to neuropathy. An excessive amount of vitamin B6 has been associated with nerve damage. If you decide to take vitamin B6, it is essential that the amount you take does not exceed more than 200mg, as if you take more than this, it can cause nerve damage.

B complex vitamins are often sold in units of 50mg, and it is probably best to start at this level and see if it is enough to alleviate some of the symptoms.

If you are concerned that some of your symptoms are being made worse by a Vitamin B deficiency, then ask your doctor to run some tests to detect whether your diet needs supplementing.

4) Magnesium

Magnesium plays an important role in transmitting impulses, allowing the muscles to relax and contract. Studies are unclear over whether the mineral could help treat diabetic neuropathy; however, it can help to effectively relieve some of the symptoms.

Magnesium can help the muscles to relax, which can help reduce cramps or spams in the lower legs. Magnesium can also help to reduce the 'restless legs' feeling that can be common in patients with neuropathy.

Several recent studies have shown a prevalence of magnesium deficiency in patients with diabetes, and some experts state that supplementing with the mineral can help reduce the risk of developing diabetes.

Magnesium is best taken along with calcium and boron, and you'll find many brands that sell this combination together to ensure that you get the right amount.

5) Alpha Lipoic Acid

A supplement that has garnered a lot of interest in recent years is alpha lipoic acid. It is believed to have many health benefits and is thought to be useful in the treatment of inflammation, Multiple Sclerosis, migraines, arterial disease and diabetes, to name a few.

Many who take this supplement believe that it reduces their symptoms, and studies have shown that it can slow the progression of neuropathy. Others report that it helps to reduce the numbness in their hands and feet.

6) Acetyl-L Carnitine

Acetyl-L Carnitine has shown promise in the treatment of diabetic neuropathy. One study showed that patients who took the supplement for a year felt a reduction in pain and there were positive changes in sensory and motor function. It is also thought to encourage nerve regeneration. However, dosages given during the study were extremely high – ranging from 1000mg – 2000mg a day, and Acetyl-L Carnitine is not readily available in doses that size.

This supplement might interfere with thyroid function, so if you are on medication for thyroid treatment, then you'll need to discuss supplementing your diet with Acetyl-L Carnitine with your doctor first.

7) Protein Powders

If you have noticed that your muscles are beginning to atrophy because of your neuropathy, then you could benefit from taking a protein powder supplement. This can be expensive; however, you could just try a basic soya protein powder, which would be sufficient to supplement your diet.

Protein is a building block for the muscles, so if you are exercising to try and reduce the chances of muscle wastage, then putting something back into the muscles is a good idea. Additionally, it might also be beneficial to supplement with amino acids; when choosing amino acids, look for a balanced supplement that contains all of the essential amino acids that your body needs. Some amino acids can act as nerve transmitters, and they can also help the muscles to recover after exercise.

8) Evening Primrose Oil

Evening Primrose Oil is often recommended for patients with neuropathy as it is believed that the GLA can help to protect the myelin sheath. Some patients find that taking regular doses of evening primrose oil can help reduce some of the symptoms such as pain and tingling.

9) Fish Oil

Fish oil acts as an anti-inflammatory and may also be helpful in reducing some of the most common symptoms of neuropathy. Other studies have shown that the oil could play a role in preventing diabetic neuropathy.

10) Vitamin E

It is believed that supplementing with vitamin E could help prevent some forms of diabetic neuropathy. Vitamin E is an antioxidant and some experts suggest that some of the complications of diabetes are caused by the oxidative stress that can be caused to the body by having high glucose levels.

Vitamin E might lower the requirements for insulin, so if you are thinking of supplementing your diet with the vitamin, then seek medical advice first.

Chapter 3) Natural Remedies for Diabetic Neuropathy

The various options described in the following chapter each have their own way of making life with neuropathy easier to manage. None of these options claim to offer a cure but they can go some way to helping to improve balance, relax muscles, and lower blood glucose.

If you are planning on trying any of the following suggestions, then ask for medical advice first to ensure that they are safe for you to try.

Also, the symptoms of neuropathy, and the treatments for them, can be a very individual thing; what works for one patient, might not be quiet so effective for another. You'll also need to find a safe and effective form of exercise that can help to boost your circulation, as increasing circulation can help reduce some of the symptoms of neuropathy.

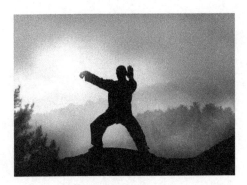

1) Tai Chi

The ancient art of Tai Chi is thought to have many benefits for people suffering from diabetes and diabetic neuropathy. Tai Chi should also be safe to practice for most people. The gentle, flowing movements are easy to follow and if you have had a period of immobility, and want to get your muscles slowly moving again without causing too much stress to your muscles and joints, then this form of exercise is ideal in many ways.

Studies have shown that Tai Chi can be helpful to patients with type 2 diabetes and it can help improve walking speed, balance, muscle strength and co-ordination.

Tai Chi has also been proven to help patients with peripheral neuropathy by increasing strength and sensation.

Tai Chi is a gentle enough exercise to do every day and it is ideal for people who haven't exercised for a while. A DVD especially aimed at diabetics is currently available for those that want an introduction to this form of gentle exercise.

Tai Chi can also help to aid relaxation and sooth the mind, so if stress is one of the things that make your blood sugar spike, then this form of moderate exercise should be suitable.

2) Reflexology

Some diabetics say that they have found that reflexology can help alleviate some of their symptoms. They feel that is helps them to get a better night's sleep and studies have shown that reflexology can reduce some of the most unpleasant symptoms of neuropathy including pain and tingling sensations.

Although this form of therapy can be self-administered, it is recommended that you see a reflexologist. Reflexology massagers and insoles are also available to buy, and these might be suitable for you if you have found reflexology to be an effective form of therapy.

3) Yoga

Yoga has been shown to help control blood sugar levels, especially in patients with type 2 diabetes. There is also some evidence that yoga asanas could help improve nerve velocity and improve nerve function in patients with sub-clinical neuropathy.

3) Acupuncture for Neuropathy

Acupuncture is a popular treatment option for people looking for pain relief. There is some limited evidence to show that acupuncture could be helpful in treating neuropathy. A study carried out by the Heidelberg School of Chinese Medicine, Heidelberg, German, involved patients with peripheral neuropathy.

It was found that acupuncture could be helpful in improving nerve conduction in patients suffering from the nerve disease.

Another study, which was entitled *Acupuncture and Neuropathy*, also showed that patients who underwent acupuncture treatments gained some relief from their symptoms and they were still reaping the benefits some six months later.

While acupuncture does not offer a cure for neuropathy patients, the studies show that it does have some major benefits.

4) Homeopathic Remedies for Neuropathy

New Era make a product designed to help patients with sciatica, neuritis or inflammatory neuropathy and neuralgia. The product consists of a combination of tissue salts; it contains Iron Phosphate, Potassium Phosphate and Magnesium Phosphate.

Some patients do find the supplement helpful in reducing nerve pain.

5) Aromatherapy

Essential oils offer many health-giving benefits, as well as helping to relax the muscles and prevent muscle cramps. For this reason they can be a useful tool when it comes to finding an effective neuropathic pain treatment and they can also work well as a lower back pain treatment, which some patients with neuropathy might experience if they have problems walking.

Studies have shown that essential oils can help to reduce peripheral neuropathic pain.

While essential oils are no means a cure, they do have the potential to offer at least some level of pain relief.

Essential oils should not be applied directly to the skin and extra care should be taken if you have sensitive skin; you'll need to blend them with some base oil such as sweet almond oil or vitamin E. Once you've mixed a blend of oils, store them in an air tight jar. It is a good idea to have some oils ready mixed so they are available whenever you need them. The oils can be applied as part of a massage either last thing at night when you need your legs to relax or at any point when you feel your muscles tensing up.

Moreover, if you are having one of those days when you are more prone to spasms and pain, then a gentle massage can go some way to helping reduce the symptoms. A regular massage is also beneficial to the circulation.

The oils can also be used in the bath, or you can buy a ready mixed blend.

NB. Some essential oils should not be used by pregnant women or patients with epilepsy. If you have any concerns about using essential oils, then seek expert advice.

Chamomile essential oil is effective at reducing back pain and will also act as a muscle relaxer. Chamomile can also help to reduce inflammation and can work as a sleep aid. Chamomile blends well with lavender essential oil, which will also aid relaxation and help ease tension.

Lemongrass essential oil is a good pain reliever and will also help to relax tired, sore muscles.

Peppermint essential oil will have a warming effect on the muscles and help the muscles to relax. It is also thought to play a role in relieving pain and can help reduce spasms.

Others oils that can be beneficial include:

- Eucalyptus
- Ginger
- Geranium Rose
- Rosemary and
- Black pepper

6) Chilli Pepper Cream

The active ingredient of chillies is capsaicin. Capsaicin is often used to treat pain and it is available in a cream form. It has been shown to reduce the discomfort of neuropathy for some patients. However, some people find it can cause irritation to the skin or redness.

Cayenne pepper is also believed to increase the circulation and it will help to warm cold lower limbs.

7) Neuropathy Formula Oil

Neuropathy Formula Oil has been created to help provide temporary relief to patients with pain and tingling in their feet; the product acts to temporarily reduce the pain. It is an all-natural product containing Frankincense & Myrrh.

8) Penetrex Cream

Penetrex cream is another all-natural product that is designed to bring relief for patients with painful conditions such as neuropathy.

It is advised to use the product at night if that is when your symptoms are worse as it might help to make the symptoms easier through the night. Moreover, it is recommended that you use the product 3-4 times a day for the first seven – ten days, and then just use the cream as necessary.

9) TENS

TENS therapy can be highly effective when it comes to managing pain. However, TENS machines aren't suitable for people with heart problems, and there are a number of other contraindications as well so they should not be used without medical consultation. Nevertheless, if you are a suitable candidate for TENS treatment then machines are readily available and they are affordably priced.

Sometimes TENS machines don't offer pain relief straight away, but if used the day before a patient can wake up relatively pain-free the next day. In addition, some people aren't comfortable with the gentle, pulsing sensation that can sometimes be felt when the TENS device is in use.

There are many different TENS devices available; each of them has different functions. Some offer programmes to help relax the muscles, which is beneficial to patients suffering from muscle spasms and cramps. They can also be used to build muscle as well, so these can be highly beneficial to patients suffering from muscle atrophy.

10) LivRelief Nerve Pain Relief Cream

This cream contains capsicum. It can be used for the nerve pain caused by diabetic neuropathy and its transdermal application means that it will get to work quickly.

It is meant to relieve the shooting, burning and stabbing pains that are common in patients with diabetic neuropathy. It can also be effective for other types of nerve pain such as a pinched nerve or shingles.

11) Pain-relieving Foot Cream

MagniLife® Pain Relieving Foot Cream is for patients with neuropathic foot pain. As well as working to reduce pain, it will also to help reduce the dry, cracked skin that can be common in diabetic patients.

12) pharMAX Nerve Pain Relief

PharMAX is a homeopathic based cream designed to help patients with nerve pain, including diabetic nerve pain. One of the main active ingredients is capsicum, but it also contains a range of other natural ingredients.

The cream can be applied four times a day if necessary.

13) Neuragen PN

Neuragen PN has been shown to be effective at reducing the pain experienced as part of diabetic neuropathy. It is another homeopathic based cream and it aims to reduce shooting, burning, stabbing and tingling pain.

14) Ultimate Neuro Neuropathy Treatment

This product uses electrotherapy so it won't be suitable for all neuropathy patients. However, this product has been developed to help address the pain caused by neuropathy

15) Diachieve Diabetic Foot Cream

This product provides temporary pain relief. It acts a topical analgesic and contains a blend of natural ingredients. It is also moisturising and rejuvenating for the skin.

16) Pain Gone Pain Relief Pen

The Pain Gone pens offer pain relief to sore joints and muscles. These can be useful for patients with neuropathy as when your walking is impaired because of neuropathy, this can make your posture awkward and cause all sorts of other aches and pains throughout your body because of the poor way that your muscles function

The pens are convenient to use and give drug free pain relief. The pen take just seconds to apply and gets to work almost straight away. It is especially good for back pain or shoulder pain, or other smaller areas where using a conventional TENS machine might be difficult.

17) Naturasil Neuropathy Rub

Naturasil Neuropathy Rub is a homeopathic product designed to provide pain relief for patients with neuropathy. The rub is suitable for all sorts of neuropathy, including diabetic neuropathy.

The product contains only plant ingredients, so this is an entirely natural product with no chemicals.

18) Pain Away Pain Relief Pen

The Pain Away Pen works in much the same way as the Pain Gone Pen and uses the principals of acupuncture. The product uses TENs therapy to reduce pain by increasing your body's natural levels of pain killing endorphins.

TENS products are not suitable for everyone, and should not be used by people who have a heart problem. Although products like these can be extremely effective for some patients, it is best to consult a doctor before proceeding with this form of pain therapy.

19) BioFreeze

Biofreeze is an effective pain reliever; its cooling effect can provide an effective form of pain relief for patients with neuropathy.

Biofreeze can be applied as a gel, spray or roll on and is especially good for use after you have done a lot of repetitive work or exercise.

If you suffer from numbness in your feet, then take care when using this product.

There are other cooling massage products available if you are unable to obtain Biofreeze.

Biofreeze can also be used by patients who suffer from joint pain and back pain. It is also good for helping to reduce the kind of pain that occurs when your muscles or joints become sore due to overuse.

21) Capsaicin Gel

Trials have found this product to be effective in reducing the pain caused by post herpetic neuralgia; patients have also found the gel to be effective at reducing the pain caused by diabetic neuropathy.

The gel can be used up to four times a day if required. However, patients must take care to wash their hands after using this product and care must be taken to not get the product near your eyes, mouth or nose in case it causes burning to sensitive areas of the skin.

Chapter 4) Exercise and Neuropathy

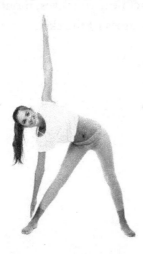

Finding suitable exercises to do when you have diabetic neuropathy can be difficult, especially if you have painful feet or a blood sugar to balance out. However, exercise had been found to reduce the pain of neuropathy and it is also believed to help slow the damage that can be caused by the nerve disease.

Ideally, you'll want to find something that is gentle for your joints and that will have minimal impact, as if you have weakened muscles then is becomes much easier to injure yourself. At the same time, you'll also want to find something that can increase blood flow and help to build some muscle.

The main aim for your exercise programme should be to:

- Build muscle and maintain muscle mass
- Improve balance
- Maintain mobility
- Mobilise your joints
- Gently stretch your muscles

It would be beneficial to see a personal instructor or to visit a gym where they can give you personalised advice for your needs. Many gyms also offer additional services such as massage therapies, and some offer complimentary therapies.

By finding a gym that can offer a combination of fitness and massage therapies, you can make it more affordable.

Once you have chosen the form of exercise you think most suitable, make sure you wear protective shoes and try wearing seamless socks as they won't rub in the same way that some footwear does.

If you need to wear orthotics to provide some additional support when you exercise, then make sure you wear insoles that are hardwearing and that are designed for diabetics.

Moreover, check your feet carefully after you have exercised for any signs of friction, rub marks, abrasions or small cuts and grazes.

Another thing you'll need to be careful of is injuries. Patients with neuropathy are more likely to develop sports injuries due to the weakened muscles in the lower legs and feet. Repetitive actions can lead to even the fittest person developing overuse injuries, and succumbing to an injury is even easier if your muscles are weak.

Moreover, if you do injure yourself, it will take much longer to heal as your weakened muscles will put a tremendous strain on your tendons, meaning the tendons won't have much of a chance to repair themselves due to the constant stress on them.

Poor circulation, and the fact that diabetics tend to take longer to heal, can mean that once you are injured, you'll face an even lengthier rehabilitation time ahead of you.

None of this is meant to put you off exercising, as there is much to be gained from it, and for some people it can be the difference between staying mobile or not. However, you do need to be clear on some of the potential pitfalls of starting a regular exercise programme.

Before you begin an exercise routine, take into consideration your limitations and discuss your plans with your doctor so they can give your some personalised advice on how to keep from injuring yourself why exercising.

Exercise can also provide an excellent means of helping to control your diabetes. However, if you have problems balancing out exercise with your insulin dose, then discuss this with your diabetes nurse so they can help you to adjust your insulin levels.

Exercises that might be suitable include:

- Cycling or an exercise bike
- Using a rowing machine or other static exercise equipment if your balance isn't very good.
- Pilates
- Yoga
- Low Impact Walking
- Indoor walking videos
- Ashtanga yoga
- Low impact exercise DVDs; Jane Fonda recently released a series of videos for older adults. They focus on low impact moves and functional exercise, so they are good if you just want to ease into some exercise without risking damage to your joints.

Exercise DVDs

Many people feel intimated by going to the gym, and it can be even more difficult when you have a disability and can't necessarily exercise in the same way that other people can.

There is an extensive range of exercise DVDs around, but not all of them will be suitable for patients with neuropathy; the aim should be to find a DVD that is low impact or that has been created for patients with limited mobility in mind.

There are exercises DVDs available for patients with diabetes, and there is one exercise programmes that has been designed for patients with neuropathy. Details of where to find these DVDs can be found in the suppliers' directory at the back of the book.

While there aren't many exercise videos around aimed at patients with neuropathy, there are several available for patients with Multiple Sclerosis. These are two different conditions, but some of the exercises in the MS DVDs do help to address some of the symptoms you might be experiencing.

The exercises on these DVDs can help improve balance and co-ordination and build strength. They can also help to improve blood flow thus improving circulation, which will beneficial to you if your hands and feet are always cold due to the neuropathy. Listed below are some of the DVDs that are available for patients with MS, and that can also be used for other conditions

1) Dahn Yoga for Multiple Sclerosis and Similar Conditions

The gentle stretches in the video are designed to aid relaxation and to improve mobility. The exercises included also aim to help reduce pain and reduce spasticity. It is also suitable for patients with other conditions such as arthritis and diabetes.

2) My MS Yoga

This yoga programme has been created by American yoga expert Baron Baptiste. The exercises on the DVD have been designed to be beneficial for patients with MS, but as they are gentle enough then they would also be okay for patients with neuropathy.

3) Yoga for MS

This DVD has been designed for patients with limited mobility. They are simple exercises that will help to maintain mobility and build strength. The exercises are simple enough for anyone to do and will help to maintain muscle tone while providing a gentle exercise routine.

4) Yoga adapted for People with Multiple Sclerosis and Other Disabilities

As well as featuring postures, the DVD also contains breathing exercises and a guided relaxation to help the body unwind and to relax tight, tense muscles.

5) Chair Yoga Program

The Chair Yoga Program is perfect for anyone keen to maintain mobility, increase their range of motion and improve their strength. The exercises have also been designed to increase circulation, reduce tension and improve day-to-day function.

Chapter 5) Coping with Night Time Pain

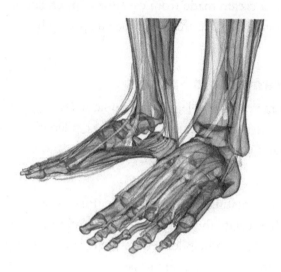

Night time can often be a distressing and depressing time for some patients with diabetic neuropathy. Some patients suffer with extreme sensitivity, and they aren't even able to tolerate the feel of the blankets against their skin. Other patients suffer badly with restless legs, while for other patients, pain can often be worse at night. The type of pain can vary from burning pains, to the feeling of electric shocks running through your feet and legs. Other patients experience painful cramps or spasms. This kind of pain is deeply unpleasant to experience and some people can find it hard to manage.

If you are troubled by night time pain, then the first step should be to talk to your neurologist. They should be able to refer you to a pain clinic where they can help you find ways to better manage your pain; they might prescribe a medication that can be taken last thing at night to help ease your discomfort, and to help you sleep better.

As stated, the pain of neuropathy might prove hard to manage for many people, but some of the other symptoms can be a little easier.

Some patients find that a cream made from cayenne pepper can be extremely helpful for nerve pain, so this could be an approach worth pursuing.

1) Night Time Cramps and Spasms

If cramps and spasms in your lower legs are a problem, try stretching out your calves before bedtime. This can help lengthen the muscles so they don't contract so badly, helping to ease the spasms.

Another method is to try rotating the ankles gently. First rotate them clockwise, and then rotate them anti-clockwise; 3-5 times each side should be enough. This can help loosen up the entire lower leg area and reduce the chance of cramps and spasms.

If you aren't currently taking medication, then try a magnesium supplement before bed. Magnesium plays a role in helping the muscles to relax, so it can help to reduce night time cramps. Magnesium sprays are also available, and these can be used for aiding sleep.

A massage lotion will help to relax your muscles last thing at night. Try a cooling massage lotion if you feel like your feet are burning, or a massage lotion to help warm the muscles if your feet feel too cold at night.

A heated massager could also be beneficial, but this is something you would have to take extreme caution with, especially if you suffer from numbness in your feet or legs. The gentle warmth can go a long way towards relaxing tight muscles, thus reducing painful cramps and spasms.

You could also try a massage cushion. These are usually designed for the back and shoulders, but you can rest your lower legs on them and get a relaxing massage for the lower leg muscles that way.

Poor circulation will contribute to the muscle cramps that you experience at night. Supplements such as Crampex are available to help ease these painful cramps. Crampex contains a form of calcium to help address any underlying calcium deficiency and also contains Niacin (Vitamin B3) to help boost the circulation to the feet.

Night splints can prove useful in keeping the muscles in the lower leg stretched out at night, which will help prevent some of the uncomfortable feelings of muscle cramps, but diabetics need to take care that the splint won't rub against their skin and cause sores or red marks. If you do decide to wear a night splint, then the health of your skin is something that should be closely monitored. Ideally, your GP should refer you to get some splints made that are suitable for you, and where possible, the straps can be lined with lambs' wool to keep them from rubbing against your skin.

Using relaxing herbs can help to reduce muscle spasms and can help to ease nerve irritation. Here are some suggestions for useful herbs:

- passionflower
- valerian
- hops
- lemon balm and
- camomile

Herbs such as Jamaican Dogwood are also believed to have powerful anti-inflammatory effects and it will also work as an anti-spasmodic.

Jamaican Dogwood is also thought to reduce nerve pain and to aid sleep.

Another technique that might help is to try a deep relaxation method last thing at night. Yoga DVDs will often have a section that will take your body through deep relaxation. This will involve relaxing and contracting each muscle in turn, helping to reduce accumulated tension in the muscles and relaxing the body.

2) Restless Legs

Many patients can find it difficult to sleep because of restless legs. There are medications that can help to manage this condition better, so get medical advice if this is a symptom you are currently struggling with. However, always try all other aids you can, before you start medication as each medication comes with it's own side effects.

Try eliminating caffeine to see if this has a positive effect on your symptoms, as caffeine can often make restless legs worse.

Ask your doctor if it would be possible to run some blood tests to check for iron deficiencies, as anaemia can often cause restless legs. It would also be a sensible idea to ask for your vitamin B12 and other B vitamin levels to be checked as well, as a lack of these vitamins can also be associated with restless legs or nerve problems.

Try to do some gentle exercises during the day, as this is thought to be beneficial to patients with restless legs and lessen the symptoms at night.

You could also try a gentle massage or some relaxation techniques to see if this helps to relieve or reduce the symptoms.

3) Night Time Sensitivity

Night Time sensitivity can prove to be a real problem for many neuropathy patients. It is possible to buy some "comfort socks" that are designed to help reduce this kind of sensitivity and they are also said to help reduce the burning pains that some patients feel.

The socks are non-elasticated so they are suitable for diabetics as they won't restrict the circulation.

4) Bed Cradles

Bed Cradles are perfect for keeping blankets off of your feet and legs. The bed cradles are especially useful for people with extreme sensitivity. Foldable bed cradles are available for purchase so they don't have to take up too much space when they are not in use.

5) Magnetic Leg Wraps

Studies have shown magnetic leg wraps to be beneficial for patients suffering from the discomfort of restless legs syndrome. Patients using these wraps have experienced a reduction in symptoms, such as tingling.

The wraps are also suitable for swollen legs, leg ulcers, cramp, and other lower leg problems.

6) Chillow Pillow

If you have ever experienced the burning feeling that makes sleep impossible, then you might benefit from using a chillow pillow. Many people used them to help keep cool during the long, hot summer nights; however, they can also be used to cool down any area of the body that gets too hot, and will help to make your limbs more comfortable.

Gel cooling pads and mattresses are also available and are designed to help you get a better night's sleep.

If you have numbness in your feet, then get some medical advice before using this product.

Chapter 6) Control your Glucose Levels

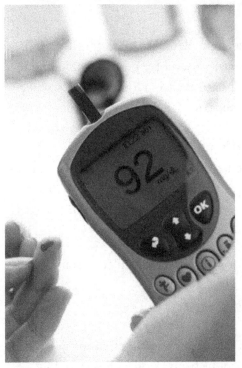

The one thing that is key to preventing diabetic neuropathy is tight glucose control. If you already have neuropathy, then getting control of your glucose levels is the best thing you can do to try and prevent further damage to the nerves.

This book cannot tell you how exactly to control your glucose levels because everyone's insulin requirements will be different and everyone will have different activity levels and eat a different diet. However, these are all things that will influence you blood sugar levels.

If you are struggling to control your glucose levels or if you find that different factors make your blood sugars harder to control at times, then you'll need to speak to your diabetes nurse.

If your diet is a problem, your diabetes nurse can refer you to a dietician to help any issues there. Stress is also another factor that you'll need to take into account. Anxiety can make your blood sugars run too low, which in turn can lead to a high blood sugar, and stressful events such as an argument could make your blood sugars spike. Getting on top of any stress issues that may adversely affect your blood sugars is crucial to helping your diabetes control.

While this book cannot give individual advice, here are a few guidelines that can help maintain steady glucose levels.

1) A Good Breakfast

Begin the day the right way. Slow release carbohydrates will help your blood sugars stay even throughout the morning and will stop you wanting to snack part way through the day.

Ideal breakfasts that will maintain your blood sugar all morning include porridge, granary toast, rye breads and muesli.

2) Lunchtime Foods

Finding healthy lunchtime foods can often be a challenge for diabetics, especially with the prevalence of snack meals. The problem with these types of foods is that they are often high in sugar, fat and unrefined carbohydrates – not the ideal diabetic diet. Ideal lunch foods include sandwiches made from granary bread or crisp breads, wholemeal pasta, bean based soup, or baked potatoes. All of those foods will provide slow release carbohydrates and give you a constant stream of energy while maintaining your blood sugar level.

Meals should also be served with protein such as meat or fish, as this will help to steady your blood sugar as well.

3) Evening Meals

Evening meals can be based on wholemeal rice, potatoes, pasta, quinoa, bulghar wheat, barley or pulses. All of these foods will help to keep your blood sugar from spiking and will help to curb your appetite.

Foods such as fruit, oatcakes or a small piece of dark chocolate make good snacks for in between meals.

4) Stress

Stress is something you must get a grip on if you want to control your blood sugars. Meditation techniques, yoga and Tai Chi can all help to aid relaxation and control stress.

5) Low Blood Sugar

In order to avoid high blood sugars, you'll want to learn how to manage your low blood sugar levels, as hypoglycaemia will often lead to hyperglycaemia, as your blood sugar will surge to compensate for running low.

If you don't know what triggers your lows, then keep a diary and see if there is a pattern. If you still find it difficult to determine what causes your blood sugar to fall too low, then speak to your diabetes nurse, as they will be able to better understand the peaks and pits in your blood sugar. Sometimes it can just be a case of adjusting insulin, other times it might be that you are on the wrong type of insulin.

6) Exercise

Chapter four discussed the importance of exercise and how it can help to relieve some of the symptoms of diabetic neuropathy. However, exercise can be beneficial for both neuropathy and diabetes.

Regular exercise will help to keep your glucose levels under control and help you to avoid spikes in your blood sugar. Exercise will also aid your circulation, which could help to ease some of your diabetic neuropathy symptoms, such as tingling. Due to the better control that exercise will give you over your blood sugar levels, this is another way of pro-actively working towards reducing the symptoms of your diabetic neuropathy.

7) Sleep

It is easy to underestimate the power of sleep and the affect it can have on your blood sugar, however, not getting enough sleep can also play havoc with your blood sugar levels.

If your body feels stressed, as it will when you've not had enough rest, your body will release a hormone called cortisol to help it cope. This hormone can cause a surge in your glucose levels. One bad night's sleep is unlikely to do too much harm; however, if the lack of sleep continues over a long period of time, then it can start to impact on your blood sugar control.

If you have pain at night and this is keeping you awake, this is another reason to discuss some of the best medication for neuropathic pain, with your doctor. Finding a suitable treatment for neuropathic pain will enable you to get a much better night's sleep and will enable you to control your blood sugars much easier.

8) Keep a Food Diary

One effective way of gaining control of your blood sugars is to keep a food diary. This is especially important if you have recently been diagnosed as diabetic and aren't used to paying so much attention to your diet.

It can be far too easy to snack on things without being conscious of it, especially if you are busy or distracted. Keeping a food diary will provide you with a clear record of everything that you eat. You can then compare your food dairy with the blood glucose diary and you'll see clearly which types of foods are making your blood sugars spike. It is not always chocolate that makes your blood sugar spike; it could be your love of starchy foods. Once you know where you are going wrong with your diet, it is much easier to fix it – and you'll be rewarded with better glucose levels.

9) Hormones

If you are female, then surges of hormones throughout the monthly cycle can also provide another challenge when it comes to managing your blood sugars.

If your estrogen levels are out of balance, then this can cause your blood sugars to soar or it can also make your blood sugars go the other way and run too low. Either way, this is another issue that will need addressing if you want to maintain optimal blood sugar control, so if you find balancing out your blood sugar levels difficult and the difficulty balancing out your glucose levels coincides with the surges in your hormonal cycle, speak to your diabetes nurse or consultant about how to manage this.

It is clear that avoiding high blood sugar is the best way to prevent the painful and sometimes disabling condition of diabetic neuropathy. The above tips will help you to make better food choices, but don't be tempted to change your diet too radically or adjust your insulin without speaking to the person responsible for your care.

Chapter 7) Foot Care

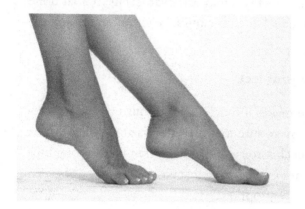

Due to the lack of sensation that many patients with diabetic neuropathy suffer from, it is essential to take care of your feet in order to avoid anything that could lead to ulceration, infection or worse. This chapter shares some advice on keeping your feet healthy.

1) Check your Feet Daily

Don't leave anything to chance and ensure that you check your feet daily for any marks, cuts or abrasions. If you notice anything that concerns you, then discuss it with your doctor. It doesn't matter how minor it might seem, even a small abrasion can lead to infection if you are not careful.

2) Bath Your Feet Daily

It's best to bathe your feet separately so you can give yourself some time to check your feet carefully. Add some tea tree oil to your water, as this is known for keeping infections at bay, and can be effective at preventing fungal infections that diabetics can be prone to.

Moreover, add some salt to the water as well. Salt is known for preventing infection and can also reduce inflammation.

Make sure you dry your feet carefully afterwards; ensure that none of the skin on your feet is left damp and take extra care to dry between your toes.

Careful not to burn your feet

The lack of sensation makes it much easier to burn the skin on your feet. Before bathing, make sure that the water is at a tolerable heat, or get someone to check it for you. Diabetic skin takes a long time to heal once it becomes injured or damaged, so doing your best to prevent damage is the best option.

3) Apply some Moisturiser

A good moisturiser is essential for avoiding dryness, which can lead to cracking of the skin, especially in diabetics, who are more prone to dry skin.

Gehwol make a range of foot creams, all of which are suitable for diabetics. If you are prone to cold feet, then look out for their foot warming cream. You'll find a list of supplies for these products in the back of the book.

4) Choose Footwear Carefully

Many people dread buying new foot wear, but this can be a special concern for diabetics. New footwear can cause friction or pressure that your feet will be unaccustomed to. This can soon lead to an ulcer or abrasions if it goes unchecked.

Check your feet extra carefully when you are breaking in new shoes, or buy some shoes that are designed especially for diabetics. You'll find a list of suppliers later on in this book.

5) Cut your Nails Straight

It is advisable that you get a chiropodist to cut your nails so they can check your feet over at the same time in case they notice any areas of concern that you might not be aware of. However, if you do decide to cut your own nails, then cut them straight so they don't catch against your socks.

As a diabetic, in some countries you are entitled to receive chiropody care free of charge. If not, you'll need to find a private chiropodist. It is recommended that you see a chiropodist every six months, or sooner if you develop any problems with your feet, such as corns or hard to cut nails.

6) Avoid Fungal Infections

Diabetics can be more prone to fungal infections. You can help to prevent this by drying your feet carefully after you have washed them and using an anti-fungal talcum powder. You can also buy anti-fungal products to paint on your toenails to help keep them free from fungus.

7) Go for Your Diabetic Checks

When you attend a diabetic clinic, they should check your feet for any potential problems. However, more often than not clinics are just asking patients if they have recently had their feet checked. If you haven't, make sure that your diabetes consultant is aware of this so that they can carry out an examination and refer you to a chiropodist if needed.

Moreover, if you have concerns over the health of your feet, explain this to your diabetes consultant

Chapter 8) Orthotics and Footwear

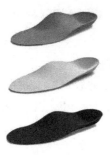

If you have developed problems with your walking due to your diabetic neuropathy, then it might be suggested that you wear orthotics to make your walking easier.

Wearing orthotics can act as shock absorbers when you walk and help to counteract problems such as pronation, which can be caused by muscle weakness.

There is a vast range of orthotics available. However, it is best for diabetics not to buy off-the-peg orthotics. If the orthotics are not designed specifically for you, then they can have a tendency to dig into the feet, cause friction against the skin, or cramp the toes up too close to the top of the shoe, causing them to rub.

As diabetics know, the slightest abrasion can go on to develop into something much more serious, so when it comes to getting orthotics, they need to be bespoke and made to accommodate your own personal needs.

There are few ways of getting orthotics that are perfect for you. The first way is to ask your GP for a referral to the local hospital, where there should be an orthotist available, who can examine your feet, suggest suitable orthotics for your needs, and order them for you. You'll then have to go back in a few weeks to have them fitted.

If you are under the care of an orthopaedic consultant, and your GP has not offered to refer you to get some orthotics made, then ask if it is possible for the Consultant to write you a referral letter. You'll be sent an appointment with an orthotist, and they will be able to help you from there.

The other option is to pay for some custom made orthotics yourself. This can be very expensive, but the quality is usually high, and it really is a case of getting what you pay for.

Some sports shops offer gait analysis and can give basic advice on orthotics, however, your best option is one of three suggestions listed above, as orthotics might need to be made in a material designed not to rub against your feet, and this can be hard to obtain without going to a specialist.

1) Therapy Socks/Neuropathy Socks
Socks for peripheral neuropathy or therapy socks were created to help give peripheral neuropathy patients a reduction in their symptoms. The socks work by helping to improve the microcirculation; it is known that poor circulation can make the symptoms of neuropathy worse.

The therapy socks are available in three different types: relaxed fit, comfort fit and slim fit. The company that supplies the socks are based in the United States, but they do ship internationally.

2) Diabetic Socks
Diabetic socks don't have seams to help avoid blisters forming on the feet. Some socks are also designed so that they control excessive moisture, which could give rise to fungal infections.

Diabetic socks should also come without elastic around the cuffs so that they are non-constricting. They should also be designed to help keep the feet warm, thus helping to aid circulation.

These socks are readily available from online retailers and come in a range of colours.

Socks for neuropathy pain are also available and you'll find details of where to get these in the suppliers' directory at the back of the book.

3) Diabetic Shoes

The range of designs for diabetic shoes is somewhat limited. However, these have been created to help avoid rubbing against the skin so they are seam free. They can be bought as shoes, trainers and boots; some suppliers offer a bespoke service.

4) Diabetic Insoles

It is also possible to buy diabetic insoles. The insoles are seam free to help avoid friction that could soon turn into blisters or ulcers. However, if they are not exactly the right size, or if they catch against your skin because the shape isn't quite suitable for your needs, then this, too, can cause friction. When it comes to insoles, it is best to get them custom made.

Chapter 9) Maintaining Dexterity

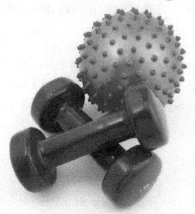

If your neuropathy progresses, then there is the possibility that you could develop muscle wasting in your hands. You might also experience some tightening in the tendons, and all of this can begin to make maintaining your dexterity difficult.

If this is a problem for you, then your first step should be to speak to your GP or neurologist. They'll be able to refer you to an occupational therapist, who can suggest gadgets to make managing everyday tasks easier.

If you are finding work difficult because you need to use your hands for typing or using a till, then again, an occupational therapist will be able to advise you on the type of products that are available to help. For instance, you might need a custom made splint to hold your hand in a better position when you type, or you might need some splints to prevent the tendons in your hands from tightening up while you sleep.

If you are struggling to stay in work because you need to do a repetitive action such as typing, then voice activated software can be an option for you.

The software does take a bit of getting used to – and you can expect plenty of typos when you first start to use it – but once the software begins to recognise your voice and the way you say things, it gets much easier.

If you don't want to go to the expense of buying software, then there are a few apps available that can be downloaded free of charge or on some versions of Windows, voice recognition software is already included.

Try searching your computer to see if this option is included, as dictating your work rather than typing will take an awful lot of stress away from the hands. Even if you just use a computer for leisure work, the voice software still works well at assisting you to complete your computer tasks without causing pain in your hands.

Voice software is also particularly good if you have developed pain in your shoulders or forearms due to the weakness in your hands. This will happen because as your hands weaken, the shoulders and forearms will be forced to work much harder, and it is a stress that they just can't cope with.

Another thing to consider if you are struggling to stay in work is the Access to Work Scheme. This is a small Government scheme that gives grants to disabled people to enable them to keep working.

The grants can be used to pay for the additional equipment that you might need in order to keep your job or a disabled person can obtain a grant to allow them to pay for a care worker to help them do the things they can no longer do. For instance, if you can't drive to work anymore, you might be able to get a grant to pay for a care worker to drive you there.

The grants are also available for self-employed people, so don't feel that just because you might not be able to do some of the things you once did, that there aren't options out there for you. At the back of the book, you'll find some information that will help you to find out more about Access to Work Grants.

If you aren't currently experiencing any muscle loss, but are concerned how the muscle atrophy related to neuropathy might affect you, then you need to be aware that there are many products that are available to help you to maintain muscle in your hands and to help you gently stretch your fingers to reduce the chances of the tendons tightening up too much. There is a stockists' directory at the back of the book if you need to purchase any of the items listed in this chapter.

Remember to gently warm your hands and wrist up before using any of the products detailed; perhaps start by circling your wrists a few times to warm them up. When you've finished, carefully stretch your fingers and wrists out afterwards to reduce tightness.

Also, build the repetitions up slowly so that you don't over work your muscles or tendons.

1) Mobilis Hand Putty

Mobilis hand putty is available in three different strengths and is ideal for helping to both strengthen your grip and to stretch the tendons. You can use the putty just by gently squeezing it in your hands. If you have any particular areas of muscle wasting, then you can concentrate on those areas.

When using the putty, rest the hand you are working on your leg, as this will avoid putting too much stress on the working hand and help to avoid overworking the muscles.

2) Grip Strengtheners

These are designed to increase the strength in the hands and forearm. They are easy to use and easy to store, so they are ideal if you are looking for a practical way of exercising your hands.

3) Dyna-Gel Therapy Balls

These balls come in four different colours; each colour represents a different resistance level. They are good for building strength in the hands and fingers without working the muscles too hard.

4) Gripmaster hand and finger exerciser

The hand and finger exerciser by Gripmaster has been created to increase dexterity and endurance in the hands and fingers. This is particularly good for people who find that their hands get tired quickly, especially when doing repetitive tasks, such as chopping vegetables.

As well as improving hand strength, they also serve to increase strength in the wrists and forearm.

5) Fitness Mad Strong Grip Hand Exerciser

This egg-shaped product helps to strengthen the hands, wrists, forearms and fingers. It can also be used as a rehabilitation tool and it aids hand co-ordination as well.

6) FlexEx Hand Exerciser

The FlexEx Exercise wraps around the fingers and provides resistance while you're carrying out exercises. It has been designed to exercise the fingers, hands and forearms and will help to gradually strengthen the muscles.

7) Handmaster Plus

This product comes in three different strengths: firm, medium or soft. As well as strengthening the muscles of the hand, the

Handmaster Plus also acts to stimulate blood flood and stimulate the peripheral nerves. This exercise device is ideal if you are losing muscle in your hands, as it works to build strength in the muscles that are responsible for opening and shutting the hand.

8) NRS Eggsercizer

This egg-shaped resistance hand exerciser will help to strengthen your grip, improve the functioning of the hand, and improve your circulation and dexterity.

The exerciser can also be used to help with RSI or Carpal Tunnel Syndrome.

9) Planet Waves Dynaflex Gyro hand Exerciser

The Gyro Hand Exerciser is designed to exercise the hand and lower arm area. They also work to build endurance, which is especially beneficial for patients with neuropathy who find that their hands get tired quickly.

This product also helps to build hand speed. An alternative to this product is the PowerBall, which works in a similar way, and is also beneficial to patients with RSI or Carpal Tunnel Syndrome.

In addition to the products mentioned above, you might also find that wrist supports or splints become necessary to help take some of the stress off of the hand muscles if they have become weakened by neuropathy.

These can be custom made for you. Your doctor can refer you to an occupational therapist or hand specialist to get some splints.

Chapter 10) Neuropathy Formulas

If you have ever searched the Internet in the hope of finding an effective treatment for your neuropathy or the neuropathic pain that comes with it, you'll no doubt have discovered some of the many neuropathy support formula capsules or nerve support formulas for neuropathy that are available. A neuropathy treatment formula is easy to find and most companies will ship worldwide if you choose to order one of the formulas offered online. However, there are a few things you'll need to take into consideration before buying.

Due to the fact that everyone reacts differently to supplements, and that readers of this book are likely to be on various other medications, there will be no recommendations for specific formulations. However, here are a few observations about the products.

There are mixed opinions on neuropathy formulas. Some people assert that some of the products are overpriced and advise that it is best to compare the products with the cost of buying the individual vitamins. Another important thing to take into consideration is the amount of each vitamin/supplement included in the product and how they compare with supplements that can be bought separately.

There are many positive reviews about the nerve formulas and people do find that the formulas do have a positive impact on their symptoms; one benefit of taking formulas is that it means not having to take numerous separate vitamin supplements so it can make it easier to maintain a nutritional support regimen.

If you do decide to proceed with using a neuropathy formula, then ideally you'll want one with B complex vitamins, Acetyl L- Carnitine and Methylcobalamin.

Some products also contain ginkgo biloba as it has been shown to improve circulation. However, gingko biloba can interact with medications such anti-convulsants, anti-depressants, blood pressure medication and blood thinning medication.

Gingko can also interact with anti-diabetic medication, thus decreasing insulin levels.

These are just some of the possible interactions with other medications that you may be on to control your blood sugar levels, to thin your blood, lower blood pressure or to ease pain.

If you are considering taking a formula, ask your doctor or neurologist to review the ingredients before purchasing to ensure it will not interact with any medication you are currently being prescribed.

Chapter 11) Other Types of Neuropathy

Although diabetic neuropathy is one of the most common types of neuropathies, there are many types of non-diabetic peripheral neuropathy. In fact, there are more than 100 different types of non-diabetic neuropathy and many different causes for them. Common types of neuropathy include polyneuropathy and mononeuropathy. Inflammatory neuropathies, such as neuritis, are not uncommon and there are also hereditary forms of the disease, such as Hereditary Motor Sensory Neuropathy. Neuropathy can also be a chronic inflammatory disorder and is known as Chronic Inflammatory Neuropathy or Chronic inflammatory demyelinating neuropathy – a condition where the myelin sheath that insulates the nerves is affected. This type of neuropathy is treated by using immune system therapy.

There are also entrapment neuropathies such as Carpal Tunnel Syndrome; Bell's palsy is another type of neuropathy.

Non-diabetic peripheral neuropathy causes

Other causes of neuropathy include:

-   Vitamin deficiencies, such as a diet lacking in B12
-   Too much of some vitamins, such as B6
-   Cancer treatment
-   Nerve injury
-   Excessive alcohol intake
-   Regular contact with some chemicals, such as arsenic, mercury or lead

The rest of this chapter will explore some of the other different types of neuropathy that you might not be so familiar with.

1) Carpal Tunnel Syndrome

Carpal Tunnel Syndrome is relatively common among diabetics. Symptoms of this type of neuropathy include pain, numbness and tingling; you might also notice pain in your forearm. People who carry out repetitive activities are more likely to develop this condition.

Treatment usually involves anti-inflammatories, exercises and splints. Patients with severe symptoms might need to undergo surgery.

2) Hereditary Motor Sensory Neuropathy

Hereditary neuropathies don't get an awful lot of attention in the media. However, these types of neuropathy are quite common. The most common type of hereditary neuropathy is a type called Charcot Marie Tooth.

The symptoms of Charcot Marie Tooth often don't come noticeable until a patient reaches their teenage years. Symptoms include muscle wasting in the arms and legs, a lack of muscle strength, absent reflexes, tingling, problems walking, muscle cramps and problems with co-ordination.

As with other neuropathies, it is more a matter of dealing with the symptoms, as there is no cure as of yet. If you have this type of neuropathy, you might be prescribed some medication to control symptoms such as pain and the tingling sensations.

You might also be given splints or orthotics to help aid your walking, and physiotherapy might also be helpful.

3) Bell's Palsy

Bell's palsy is a temporary paralysis of the facial muscles and stems from a dysfunction of the cranial nerve. In Bell's palsy, only one side of the face is usually affected.

Bell's palsy tends to be short lived and many patients will recover within a few weeks. Medications include corticosteroids, physiotherapy, and in some cases, surgery may be necessary.

This type of nerve problem can be as a result of a stroke, or it is sometimes related to a virus, however, often Bell's palsy has no known cause.

4) Mononeuropathy

If a patient has mononeuropathy, it means that just one nerve has been affected. Trauma and infection can often cause this type of neuropathy.

Most often, mononeuropathy is caused by nerve compression. This can lead to conditions such as Carpal Tunnel Syndrome.

5) Polyneuropathy

Polyneuropathy affects more than one nerve in the body and will often affect many different nerves at the same time. It is sometimes referred to as chronic inflammatory neuropathy and it is a form of inflammatory peripheral neuropathy.

The symptoms of this type of neuropathy are the same as other types of neuropathy and will include symptoms such as muscle weakness, poor co-ordination, burning pains and pins and needles.

Polyneuropathy can be a result of diabetes or excessive drinking. Treatments are limited to controlling pain and physiotherapy to help the patient keep mobile.

6) Multifocal motor neuropathy

Another form of neuropathy is multifocal motor neuropathy. Much like other forms of neuropathy, the symptoms of this form of neuropathy are similar to that of peripheral motor neuropathy or chronic peripheral neuropathy in that the muscles mostly affected are the hands and the legs.

Multifocal motor neuropathy can cause wasting in the hands and the feet, eventually leading to a foot drop or weakened muscles in the wrist.

Where this type of neuropathy differs from other forms of the disease is that the symptoms can worsen significantly during colder periods. Patients with this type of neuropathy can also experience other neurological problems, such as twitching. However, multifocal motor neuropathy does not affect the sensory nerves, so feeling in the extremities should remain normal.

Unlike other neuropathies, multifocal motor neuropathy can be treated and patients who seek early intervention should be able to avoid a significant disability.

7) Chemicals and Neuropathy

People who work with chemicals can suffer from toxic neuropathy.

Exposure to some types of chemicals can cause the symptoms of peripheral neuropathy. For instance, some dentists find themselves suffering from the symptoms of neuropathy due to the exposure to chemicals such as mercury.

Moreover, farmers can also experience the symptoms of nerve damage because of the chemicals that they are exposed to on an everyday basis. People working regularly with industrial chemicals can also be vulnerable to neuropathy.

Using paints that contain high levels of led can also lead to a person experiencing symptoms of neuropathy.

Patients undergoing chemotherapy can develop peripheral neuropathy as well. Like other types of neuropathy, chemotherapy induced neuropathy is hard to treat and it can be some time before the symptoms begin to subside.

Patients with cancer can also be susceptible to this type of nerve damage.

Chapter 12) Draw up an Action Plan

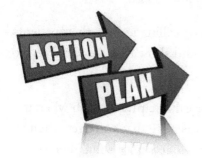

Coping with a condition that has been deemed incurable can be a daunting prospect, but as this book shows, there are many effective ways of being able to manage the symptoms of your condition.

There's nothing worse than feeling like you can't help yourself, so drawing up an action plan can help keep you motivated to find ways of dealing with your condition. When confronting neuropathy, it is best to deal with the symptoms one by one.

When it comes to drawing up your own personal action plan, there are some main points your plan should focus on:

- Diabetes control
- Exercise
- Foot Care
- Pain Relief
- Managing night time discomfort
- Addressing problems with balance

The previous chapters help to provide guidelines so you, as the patient, are aware of the many options available to you. By addressing each of these issues one by one, you can come up with a plan to make your everyday life more manageable.

Once you've come up with a plan, don't be frightened to approach your GP or consultant with your plan and don't be afraid to ask for the help you need to put your plan into action.

The majority of doctors are only too willing to help their patients – especially when they are proactive and show that they are keen to help themselves.

If you find that your family doctor isn't helpful enough when it comes to accessing the care and assistance that you need, then speak to your consultant. If either of those two options fail, then see another GP who will help.

There are plenty of ways of achieving pain relief and pain control, which for many patients can be the most difficult part of their neuropathy, so there is no reason why you should not get the access to the care you need.

Likewise, if your neuropathy has left you disabled or with limited use of your hands or legs, ask to see a physiotherapist or see one privately, and make sure that you get the care you need.

If you need adaptations around the house, then ask to be put in touch with an Occupational Therapist or if you are working and struggling to stay in work because of your neuropathy, then go to your local Job Centre and ask to see a Disability Employment Advisor; they can give you some advice on the types of options that are available to help disabled people stay in work. They can also offer advice on the obligations of your employer to provide adequate workplace adaptations if you need them.

None of the symptoms of neuropathy are pleasant; however, there are ways of managing most of them. Most patients with neuropathy are going to be experiencing some type of pain, so if you aren't already on medication, then speak to the person in charge of your care about this. With so many effective medications available to control nerve pain, there is no reason why you should have to live with it.

If the medication you are currently prescribed just doesn't work, or leaves you with side effects that are far worse, then don't be afraid to ask your doctor for an alternative means of pain control and push for a referral to a pain clinic if your pain isn't manageable.

If you really don't like the idea of medication – and many people don't – then try some of the more natural alternatives, such as the chill pepper creams or topical analgesics.

Don't be scared to look at alternative therapies such as reflexology or acupuncture. None of these things will offer a cure, but they can make your symptoms easier to cope with.

If muscle tightness is a problem, then adopt a light exercise programme that consists of gentle stretches and focus specifically on stretching your lower legs, ankles, wrists, fingers and hands.

Gentle stretching can help reduce the uncomfortable feelings of muscle spasms or cramps and can make your walking easier.

If your balance is an issue, then do some exercise to help improve your balance or try a balance board. Likewise, if you are losing muscle, then do your best to maintain it by introducing an exercise programme to help keep the muscles built and again, concentrate on building up the lower leg muscles and muscles in the hands and forearms.

If your blood sugars are contributing to your neuropathy, then take action to begin addressing this. Speak to your GP, diabetes consultant or diabetes nurse to help address any of the issues that cause your blood sugars to run too high.

Ask to see a dietician, as they will work with your diabetes team to help plan your diet and adjust your insulin doses accordingly.

Chapter 13) Hope on the Horizon?

With new research comes a better understanding of diabetic neuropathy and one day this will lead to more treatment options for people with this condition.

Several studies have been carried out in recent years that could offer hope in the future. One such method includes gene therapy, where researchers suggest that a single injection could help patients suffering from neuropathy.

Trials to test the feasibility of using gene therapy to treat diabetic neuropathy have been carried out, and the early results have been positive.

In other research, scientists have discovered that heat shock protein could help resolve the numbness that patients with diabetic neuropathy experience. Other studies have shown that carrying out a skin biopsy could be a quicker way of diagnosing diabetic neuropathy.

Although it might not be reported in the media very often, researchers are hard at work trying to develop new ways of diagnosing, treating and managing neuropathy.

Although none of this will help patients with diabetic neuropathy now, down the line it could lead to more effective ways of coping with the condition.

Stem Cells

Stem cells could one day be used as a treatment for diabetic neuropathy. There is already some evidence to show that it has helped to improve the symptoms of patients with hereditary forms of neuropathy and stem cell therapy has also shown promising results in the treatment of Chronic Inflammatory Demyelinating Polyneuropathy.

Stem cell therapy also offers hope for an array of other diseases as well. There is hope that stem cells could one day be used to treat diabetes itself or that stem cell therapy could be used to help paralyzed patients to walk again.

With all of the new advances in the medical world, hopefully it won't be long before researchers can find a way of helping patients to better manage their neuropathy and establish new ways of helping patients find an effective treatment for diabetic neuropathy pain.

Diabetic Neuropathy Blogs

People often go online to share their thoughts, feelings and daily battles when it comes to dealing with various health conditions. Reading other people's blogs can be both educational and inspiring, and help you to realise that there is help available.

Blogs are a brilliant way to learn from people's first-hand accounts of dealing with diabetic neuropathy and the writers often share tips that you might not have thought of on your own. On some blogs, you'll also find information on how the various medications help or hinder people, what the side effects are etc.

Here's a list of blogs you'll find helpful

Diabetes and Neuropathy

The diabetes and neuropathy blog details one person's account of coping with autonomic neuropathy. Not only that, but there is also plenty of useful information about using an insulin pump, reviews on different glucose meters and some of the latest news regarding diabetes.

This is a good all round blog for finding out about diabetic neuropathy and the ups and downs that come with it.

http://diabetes-and-neuropathy.blogspot.co.uk/

My Numb Feet

My Numb Feet tends to concentrate on some of the possible therapeutic treatments for neuropathy, such as light therapy, B vitamin supplements and other supplements that might help to nourish the nerves and reduce the symptoms of neuropathy.

http://mynumbfeet.blogspot.co.uk/

PN Resources

This useful blog is full of links and resources for patients with diabetic neuropathy; it is also extremely useful for patients with other types of neuropathy.

You'll find plenty of links to important research that details how complimentary or alternative therapies might be useful and links to information on prescription drugs.

There are also plenty of links to articles about peripheral neuropathy, diabetic neuropathy and small fibre neuropathy.

http://neuropathystory.wordpress.com/references/

The NP Mom

This blog has an interesting overview of diabetic neuropathy and lots of helpful links related to other health issues.

http://thenpmom.wordpress.com/2012/04/09/peripheral-neuropathy-feel-the-burn/

The Carpal Tunnel blog

As explained earlier in the book, diabetics can be prone to Carpal Tunnel Syndrome, an entrapment neuropathy that causes pain in the wrists, fingers and hands.

The blog shares information on the latest studies and also includes information of wrist exercises and massage techniques that patients with Carpal Tunnel Syndrome will no doubt find interesting.

http://carpaltunnelblog.blogspot.co.uk/

Carpal Tunnel Numbness

The blog goes into great detail about Carpal Tunnel Syndrome, explaining the symptoms, the causes, and some of the possible therapies to help treat this painful condition.

http://carpaltunnelnumbness.info/blog-articles/

Diabetes Mine

This blog contains a wealth of information on diabetes and how it contributes to Carpal Tunnel Syndrome. There is also plenty of information about the latest research into diabetes.

http://www.diabetesmine.com/2012/03/the-411-on-carpal-tunnel-syndrome-diabetes.html

Bell's Palsy

This blog details one woman's account of dealing with Bell's palsy. It makes an interesting and inspiring read.

http://caseofbellspalsy.blogspot.co.uk/

Informatics Bell's Palsy

This blog gives an excellent overview of Bell's palsy and its treatments, symptoms and management.

It also details how exercise, physiotherapy, surgery and complimentary treatments might be helpful for people with this condition.

http://informaticsbellspalsy.blogspot.co.uk/

Forums

There are numerous forums online that offer a wealth of information for diabetics. Many of these patients will also be coping with diabetic neuropathy, so these forums provide a great opportunity to learn from other patients with the same condition.

The online forums are friendly communities and they offer a good place to interact with other people who are experiencing the same symptoms as you.

Finding a diabetic neuropathy forum can be a lifeline for many people, especially if they are newly diagnosed with neuropathy and finding it hard to cope with the symptoms. Each of the forums listed below have helpful discussions about diabetic neuropathy.

The Diabetes Forum

The Diabetes Forum is based in the United States. There are many discussions on the forum about managing and coping with diabetic neuropathy.

http://www.diabetesforum.com/introduce-yourself/2842-diabetic-neuropathy.html

Pain Research Forum

The Pain Research Forum discusses pain in general. However, there are also useful discussions about coping with the pain of diabetic neuropathy and neuropathic pain.

http://www.painresearchforum.org/news/16669-clues-riddle-pain-diabetic-neuropathy

Diabetes Daily

The Diabetes Daily forum has information about neuropathy and there are also useful discussions about controlling your glucose levels and testing blood sugars.

You'll find information about the best times to test your blood sugars and managing your diet.

http://www.diabetesdaily.com/forum/neuropathy/65427-pre diabetic-neuropathy/

Resources

The following pages include links to resources that will help you to maintain hand and leg strength.

Exercises to help reduce hand and wrist pain, and to maintain range of motion:

http://www.health.harvard.edu/healthbeat/5-exercises-to-improve-hand-mobility-and-reduce-pain

Improve balance:

http://www.medicinenet.com/script/main/art.asp?articlekey=10245

Handmaster Plus

This video explains how to use the Handmaster plus for the best results.

http://www.youtube.com/watch?v=WMsxGfACAfo

Grip Master Hand Exercisers

http://www.gripmaster.com.au/index1.htm

This page details the NICE guidelines for pain relief for diabetic neuropathy. Neuropathic pain treatments are detailed in full on the NICE website, so if you suffer from this type of pain and are not sure what kind of treatments are available, you'll find some guidelines there that can help.

http://www.nice.org.uk/newsroom/pressreleases/press_releases.jsp?domedia=1&mid=8AE67557-19B9-E0B5-D4F86877017CCC38

Access to Work

If your diabetic neuropathy has made it difficult to stay in work and you need support to either stay in work, to start work, or to go self-employed, then you might qualify for support from the Access to Work scheme. Details are available by going to:

https://www.gov.uk/access-to-work

Sources:

Effectiveness of different benfotiamine dosage regimens in the treatment of painful diabetic neuropathy.

http://www.ncbi.nlm.nih.gov/pubmed/10219465

Winkler G, Pál B, Nagybéganyi E, Ory I, Porochnavec M, Kempler P.

2nd Department of Internal Medicine, Municipal St. John's Hospital, Budapest, Hungary

Effects of methylcobalamin on diabetic neuropathy

http://www.ncbi.nlm.nih.gov/pubmed/1324807

Yaqub BA, Siddique A, Sulimani R.

Division of Neurology, King Khalid University Hospital, Riyadh, Saudi Arabia.

A prospective, open label, 24-week trial of methylcobalamin in the treatment of diabetic polyneuropathy.

http://www.scirp.org/journal/PaperInformation.aspx?paperID=24765

Jacqueline C. Dominguez, Arlene R. Ng, Ludwig F. Damian

α-Lipoic Acid, Diabetic Neuropathy, and Nathan's Prophecy.

http://ang.sagepub.com/content/63/2/81.short

Outpatient Clinic of the Diabetic Foot, Second Department of Internal Medicine, Democritus University of Thrace, Greece.

N. Papanas, Second Department of Internal Medicine, Democritus University of Thrace, University Hospital of Alexandroupolis, 68100 Alexandroupolis.

Acetyl-L-carnitine (levacecarnine) in the treatment of diabetic neuropathy. A long-term, randomised, double-blind, placebo-controlled study.

De Grandis D, Minardi C.

Department of Neuroscience, Ospedale Civile, Rovigo, Italy.

http://www.ncbi.nlm.nih.gov/pubmed/12135119

Fish oil supplementation prevents diabetes-induced nerve conduction velocity and neuroanatomical changes in rats.

Diabetology Department, CHU Timone, 13385 Marseille Cedex 5, France.

http://www.ncbi.nlm.nih.gov/pubmed/9915901

Neuropathies: Essential Oils Show Promising Results.

http://theida.com/ew/wp-content/uploads/2010/10/Neuropathies-Essential-oils-show-promising-results-in-the-fight-against-symptoms.pdf

Suppliers' Directory

Some of these products will be readily available from high street stores; nutrition products should be available from your local health food store. In case of any difficulties finding any of the products mentioned in the book, here is a list of online suppliers.

Just search for the product on the websites listed below.

UK

Mobilis Hand Putty

http://www.completecareshop.co.uk

Grip Strengheners

http://www.physioroom.com

Gehwol Cream

Gehwol foot creams can be found in most health food store chains, or bought online. http://www.yourhealthfoodstore.co.uk

Power Ball

http://www.physioroom.com

Grip Master:

http://www.physioroom.com

Dyna-Gel Therapy Balls

http://www.fireflymobility.com

http://www.phillipsmobility.co.uk

http://www.welcomemobility.co.uk

Fitness Mad Strong Grip Hand Exerciser

http://physiowarehouse.co.uk

http://www.discount-supplements.co.uk

Flex ex hand exercisers

http://www.amazon.co.uk

Handmaster Plus

http://www.goodhealthmatters.co.uk

NRS Eggsercizer:

http://www.amazon.co.uk

Neuropathy rubbing oil can be ordered from iHerb:

http://www.iherb.com

Penetrex cream can be ordered direct from the manufacturers:

http://www.penetrex.com

PharMAX cream:

http://www.nutri-health.com/pharmax-nerve

Neuragen PN cream is hard to obtain in the UK, but can be bought from eBay.com

United States and Canada

Mobilis Hand Therapy Putty

This product is hard to get hold of in the United States. However, Thera-Flex has a similar product that can be purchased from Amazon.com.

http://www.amazon.com

Power Ball exercisers can be purchased from Wal-Mart. They are also available from eBay.com.

Dyna-Gel Therapy Balls

Dyna-Gel therapy balls can be purchased from:

http://www.amazon.com

Grip Master

http://www.dickssportinggoods.com

Grip Strengheners

http://www.chokesports.com

Flex ex hand exercisers

http://www.amazon.ca

The Handmaster Plus

The Handmaster Plus is available in the United States by going direct to the manufacturer's website. The website also contains detailed diagrams and videos on how to use the Handmaster Plus effectively.

http://www.handmasterplus.com

The NRS Eggsercizer can be bought from:

http://www.langtoninfo.com

Penetrex cream

http://www.penetrex.com

Neuragen PN

http://www.walgreens.com

http://www.cvs.com

LivRelief Nerve Pain Cream

The cream can be purchased from shoppers drug mart, Pharmasave, Rexall, Metro Pharmacy, London Drugs, Food Basics Pharmacy, Sobeys Pharmacy, Lawtons Drugs and the Freshco Pharmacy.

Australia

The Handmaster plus can be purchased from:

http://www.ergonomicsnow.com.au

http://handmasterplus.com.au

NRS Eggsercizer

The NRG Eggsercizer can be ordered from a UK-based company. If you have problems finding them; they ship worldwide.

http://www.fishpond.co.uk

The Fitness Mad Strong Grip Hand Exerciser can be obtained from:

http://www.ebay.com.au

Fitness Mad Hand Exerciser

A similar product to the Fitness Mad hand exerciser can be purchased from:

http://www.fitness-mad.com

Power Ball

A product similar to the Power Ball, can be obtained from:

http://www.physiosupplies.com.au

Grip Master

The Grip Master is available from:

http://www.gripmaster.com.au/index1.htm

Dyna Gel Therapy Balls can be brought from:

http://www.essentialaids.com

They are also available from some sellers on eBay if you are unable to obtain them any other way.

Flex Ex Hand Exerciser

http://aussiesupershop.com.au

Dahn Yoga DVDs are available from Amazon.com and Amazon.co.uk.

Leg wraps can be ordered from:

http://www.legtreatments.com

They accept payments via Credit card or PayPal and they ship worldwide.

Neuropathy socks or therapy socks

These can help bring relief to patients with chronic neuropathy. They can be ordered direct from:

http://www.therapysocks.com

The company ships worldwide and accepts payment via credit card or PayPal.

Other Products:

http://www.livrelief.com

http://magnilife.com

http://www.naturalhealthyconcepts.com

TENS Machines

TENS can be an effective form of pain treatment for many people; many patients find TENS useful for helping them cope with treating neuropathic pain and for finding relief for diabetic neuropathy.

TENS machines are available from chain stores and chemists. They can also be purchased online from physiotherapy stores or sporting goods' stores.

Bed Cradles

Bed Cradles are available from mobility aid or disability aid stores. They can also be bought from eBay or Amazon if you have problems obtaining them.

Footwear and Orthotics:

UK

Therapeutic Diabetic Insoles can be found at:

http://www.foothealthcare.com

As well as being suitable for patients with diabetic neuropathy, they can also be used for patients with Charcot foot, bunions, Metatarasalgia and Plantar fasciitis.

Diabetic Shoes

http://www.simplyfeet.co.uk

US and Canada

Diabetic insoles can be bought at:

http://www.soletech.com

They are also available from chain stores such as Wal-Mart.

http://www.footlogics.ca

Diabetic shoes

http://www.shoebuy.com

http://www.drcomfort.com/

Australia

Diabetic Insoles

http://www.footcareinternational.com

Diabetic Shoes

http://www.grundysshoes.com.au

Support Groups

It can be difficult to know where to turn when you are first diagnosed with diabetic neuropathy, and sometimes, medical care or medical knowledge can be limited, depending on the area you live in.

Likewise, suddenly being diagnosed as diabetic can be a difficult experience, especially when you have to totally change your life style in order to keep your blood sugars under control.

However, there are plenty of support groups available for patients with neuropathy and diabetes.

In this section you'll find a list of support groups.

UK

The Neuropathy Trust

The Neuropathy Trust offers support to patients suffering from neuropathy and neuropathic pain.

http:// multiscentre com Neuropathy /

The Centre for Neuromuscular Diseases

The Centre for Neuromuscular Diseases offers specialist care for patients suffering from neurological diseases, including peripheral neuropathy and chronic inflammatory peripheral neuropathy.

As well as helping people with peripheral neuropathy, they can also assist patients with hereditary forms of neuropathy.

Among the treatments offered are orthotics, occupational therapy, physiotherapy and Immunosuppressant therapy. There is also the opportunity the take part in clinical trials, if this is deemed appropriate.

Patients can access the services of the Centre, which is based in London, by asking their specialist or GP for a referral.

The website also offers a number of publications for patients with neuropathy.

http://www.cnmd.ac.uk/our_services/clinical_services/Peripheral_Nerve/General_Peripheral_Nerve_Service

US

The Neuropathy Association

The Neuropathy Association work towards finding a cure for neuropathy; the Association provides a wealth of information on chronic neuropathy treatment.

The association has also produced a DVD to help patients coping with chronic neuropathy and chronic neuropathy pain.

Details of the free DVD can be found by visiting:

http://www.neuropathysupportnetwork.org/order-neuropathy-dvd.html

The website can be found at:

http://www.neuropathysupportnetwork.org/order-neuropathy-dvd.html

Australia

If you are in search of neuropathic pain relief, then you'll find this website an ideal resource. The group is free to join and offers help and advice to people suffering from painful neuropathy.

http://neuropathic.tripod.com/

The Nerve Support Association in Australia has a lot of helpful information on Inflammatory Neuropathies, Multifocal Motor Neuropathy and Peripheral Neuropathy.

They are also carrying out useful research into neuropathic pain and acupuncture.

http://sydney.edu.au/medicine/nrf/research/index.php

The Inflammatory Neuropathy Support Group of Australia

The support group offers help and advice to patients and their carers. They also issue regular newsletters that contain a wealth of information for patients with inflammatory neuropathy, including information on how to cope with chronic pain and neuropathy.

http://www.ingroup.org.au/index.php?option=com_content&view=article&id=49&Itemid=55

Peripheral Neuropathy Support Group

http://www.ingroup.org.au/index.php?option=com_content&view=article&id=49&Itemid=55

Support Groups Canada

Calgary Neuropathy Association

The association offers support to patients with peripheral neuropathy and diabetic neuropathy. They also offer advice on coping with neuropathic pain.

http://calgaryneuropathy.com/

The Peripheral Nerve Society

Based in Canada, this site has a list of useful groups for patients suffering from peripheral neuropathy. www.pnsociety.com

Acknowledgements:

Special thanks to Dr Bonnie Gerecke for her contributions to this book.

Further Reading:

Diabetic Neuropathy

Diabetic Neuropathy, Tesfaye, Solomon and Boulton, Andrew.

Diabetic Neuropathy Gries, Friedrich and Cameron, Norman Defeat Chronic Pain Now? Ground-breaking strategies for eliminating the pain of Arthritis, Back and Neck conditions, Migraines, Diabetic Neuropathy. Argoff, Charles and Galer, Bradley.

Diabetic Neuropathy Mini Atlas, Luis Raul Lepori.

Neuropathy and Diabetes: Your Simple 10-Step Plan to Prevent Diabetic Nerve Damage. Centers for Disease Control and Prevention.

Painful Diabetic Neuropathy in Clinical Practice. Boulton, Andrew J.M. and Vileikyte, Loretta.

Neuropathic Pain. Bennett, Michael.

Pain Management

Overcoming Chronic Pain – A Self-help guide to using Cognitive Behavioral Techniques. Cole, Frances.

Mindfulness Meditations for Pain Relief: Guided Practices for Reclaiming Your Body and Your Life. Jon Kabat-Zinn.

The Simple Pain Management Guide, How to Quickly Heal, Treat and Cure Your Body Parts from Pain. Carter, Jeff.

Blood Sugar Management

Dr Bernstein's Diabetic Solution: A Complete Guide to Achieving Normal Blood Sugar Levels. Dr Richard K. Bernstein.

Think Like a Pancreas. Scheiner, Gary.

Using Insulin: Everything you need to Know for Success with Insulin. Walsh, John, Roberts, Ruth and Varma, Chandrasekhar.

Journals

Pathophysiology of peripheral neuropathy in diabetes

The following article, written by Mitra Tavakoli, MSc, Moaz Mojaddidi, MD,Hassan Fadavi, MD, and Rayaz A. Malik, MD, PhD discusses the pathophysiology and treatment of painful diabetic neuropathy.

http://www.academia.edu/295733/Pathophysiology_and_Tre atment_of_Painful_Diabetic_Neuropathy

The article also goes into great detail about neuropathic pain and gives a detailed explanation of diabetic peripheral neuropathic pain.

Advances in Neuropathic Pain, diagnosis, mechanisms, and treatments.

http://archneur.jamanetwork.com/article.aspx?articleid=784895

This journal article discusses treatment for diabetic neuropathic pain in great detail.

DVDs

Tai Chi for Diabetes

Yoga for Diabetes

Mayo Clinic Wellness Solutions for Type 2 Diabetes

Glossary

Type one diabetes

Type one diabetes is caused when the immune system destroys the insulin producing cells in the pancreas. This results in an inability to control blood sugar levels, so insulin has to be given in injection form.

Type two diabetes

Type two diabetes is more common in middle-aged adults. It is common among people who are overweight and it could be considered a "lifestyle" disease.

Filament test

Filament testing assesses the ability of a patient to feel sensation. These kinds of tests are often carried out on patients with diabetic neuropathy to test the sensation in the feet.

Nerve conduction

Nerve conduction tests will show how fast the nerves send electrical signals to the muscles.

The tests can cause some discomfort as it involves having electric impulses sent through the body. These types of tests are often carried out to assess neurological diseases.

Electromyography

Electromyography testing is used to assess how well the nerves work and how well the nerves send messages to the muscles.

Motor function

Motor function refers to movement. When motor function is impaired, it can affect the way a person walks, balances and co-ordinates. Problems with motor function can be common in patients with neuropathy.

Sensory function

Sensory function refers to how well your body can sense heat, touch, pain etc. Sensory function is often impaired in patients with diabetic neuropathy, which means they can be prone to injuries that go un-noticed due to the lack of feeling.

Lack of feeling can lead to serious complications if patients don't carry out regular foot checks.

Anti-depressants

Drugs used to treat the symptoms of depression. There are many different drugs available, commonly prescribed anti-depressants include Sertraline or Zoloft and Prozac or Fluoxetine.

The tricyclic form of anti-depressants are often prescribed to help treat nerve pain.

Anti-epilepsy

Anti-epilepsy drugs are used to reduce and prevent epileptic fits. They can also be used to help control muscle spasms.

Pain control

Pain control can come in the form of drugs, local anaesthetics or nerve blocks.

Pain killers

Drugs used to help relieve a patient's discomfort. They can come in capsule, tablet, liquid or injection form. Pain killers are sometimes applied in the form of topical patches.

Neurontin

Also known as gabapentin, Neurontin is an anti-epileptic drug and is also used to alleviate nerve pain.

Lyrica

Lyrica, or Pregabalin is another anti-convulsant drug. It can also be used to control nerve pain.

Tramadol

Is an opioid analgesic used for providing pain relief in neurological disorders. It can also be used to treat restless legs syndrome.

Lidocaine

Lidocaine has lidocaine hydrochloride as its main ingredient. The drug is commonly used as an aesthetic.

Opioids

Opioids are prescribed to patients suffering from moderate-severe pain. They are commonly prescribed for patients suffering from chronic pain and they have a morphine- like effect on the body.

Dramadol

Dramadol is a pain relieving drug. It is known as *Tramadol* in some countries, such as the US.

Benfotiamine

Benfotaimine is a fat soluble form of vitamin B1. It is thought to be better absorbed by the body and is believed to be helpful to patients with diabetes and neuropathy.

Methylcobalamin

Methylcobalmin is a potent form of vitamin B12. It is better absorbed by the body. Research has shown it to help patients with peripheral diabetic neuropathy.

Alpha Liopic Acid

Alpha Liopic Acid works as an antioxidant in the body. It has been shown to be useful in the treatment of diabetic neuropathy.

Acetyl-L Carnitine

Acetyl-L Carnitine is an amino acid. It is thought to help with fat metabolism. Studies have shown it to be a useful treatment for diabetic peripheral neuropathy.

Acetyl-L Carnitine is a useful aid for painful diabetic neuropathy, as it is an effective pain relief treatment.

Evening Primrose Oil

Evening primrose oil is extracted from the plant. Evening primrose oil contains GLA, which is believed to protect the myelin sheath from damage.

It is often taken by patients with MS and it is also thought to be beneficial to diabetics.

Tai Chi

Tai Chi is a form of martial arts. Tai chi is Chinese in origin and it is thought to have many health benefits.

Spasticity

Spasticity is common in patients with neurological disorders. It refers to the stiffness and tightness in the muscles that can result in a muscle spasm.

Nerve velocity

Nerve velocity measures how quickly the electrical signals are sent to the peripheral nerves.

Sub-clinical neuropathy

Patients with sub-clinical neuropathy will show abnormal test results, but will not yet be experiencing the symptoms of neuropathy.

Reflexology

An alternative treatment. Reflexologists believe that it is possible to treat different areas of the body by massaging different areas of the feet. It is believed that each individual area of the foot represents a different part of the body.

Yoga

A series of postures that have a powerful effect on the mind and the body. Yoga is an ancient art and it is believed to be beneficial to the muscles, joints and nervous system.

Magnesium

A mineral that aids healthy heart function, relaxes the muscles and allows the proper sending of nerve impulses. It is best taken with calcium.

Restless Legs

A condition that can cause uncontrollably twitching and other feelings of discomfort in the legs. It is more common at night.

Orthotics

An insole that is fitted inside the shoe to help alleviate problems such as pronation, muscle weakness or weak arches.

Carpal Tunnel Syndrome

A condition that causes pain in the hands. It is a form of neuropathy, and it is often more common in patients with diabetes. It can be caused by repetitive actions, such as typing.

Hereditary Motor Sensory Neuropathy

Hereditary neuropathies often becomes symptomatic during the childhood or teenage years. This is a genetic disorder that affects the peripheral nerves.

Polyneuropathy

Polyneuropathy affects more than one nerve. Polyneuropathy can be a complication of diabetes. It can also be caused by other factors and it is common in patients with alcoholism.

Mononeuropathy

In cases of mononeuropathy, only one nerve is affected.

Credits:

© gege2812 - Fotolia.com

© jtanki Fotolia.com

© Africa Studio - Fotolia.com

© ingridat - Fotolia.com

© evgenyb - Fotolia.com

© falaterphotog - Fotolia.com

© filipw - Fotolia.com

© Aliaksei Luskin - Fotolia.com

© SCHMaster - Fotolia.com

© marinini - Fotolia.com

Index

Printed in April 2023
by Rotomail Italia S.p.A., Vignate (MI) - Italy